Siegfried Gursche

Juicing –
for the Health of it!

Release the Healing Power of Plants for Optimum Health

alive books

Vancouver
Canada

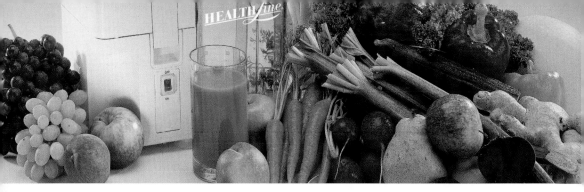

Contents

All About Juice

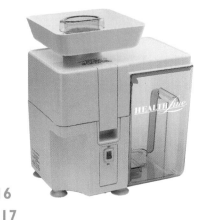

Recipes

Recipes

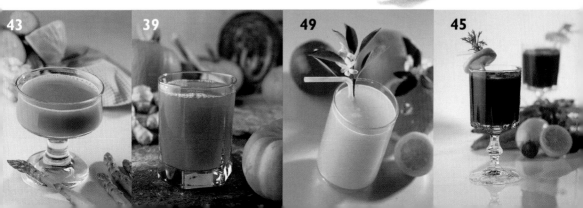

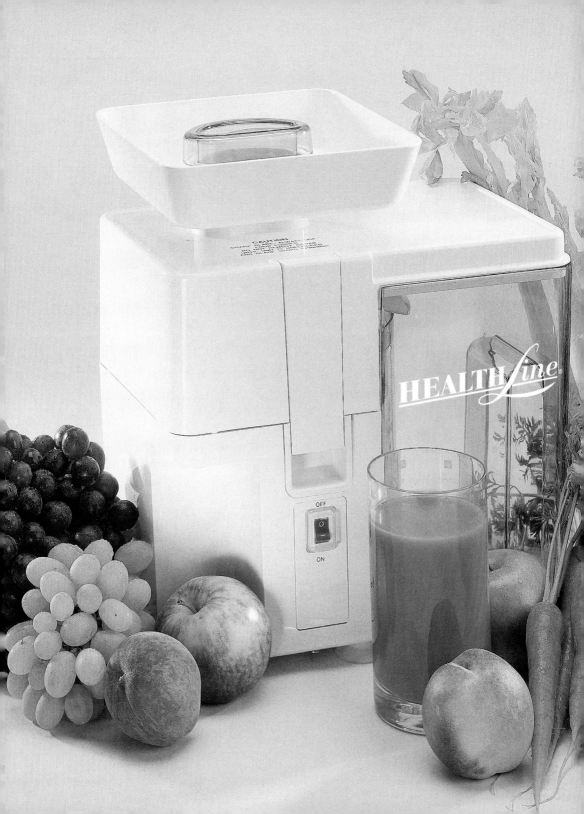

All About
Juice

Raw juices are for everybody. Unlike cooked food, the nutrients
found in juices retain their natural molecule structure, which
the body recognizes instantly and puts to work immediately–
without a lengthy digestion time. You are ingesting live food,
that's why you feel better! I guarantee it, no matter what your
state of health.

– Siegfried Gursche

Every morning I have a tall glass of freshly pressed juice before breakfast. However, when I travel this is not always possible. Do I feel the difference? You bet I do! Starting my day with food full of vitamins, minerals and enzymes–especially in a concentrated form like freshly extracted juice–is like tapping into a power-house of energy. Not only does it wake me up, it keeps me going throughout the day.

Fruits and vegetables have been recognized throughout the history of man as a natural source of valuable nutrients, essen-

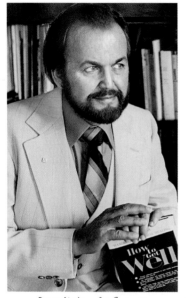

*Paavo Airola
(1918 - 1983)*

tial to health and well-being. At the beginning of creation God said, "Behold, I have given you every plant yielding seed; it shall be food for you," (Genesis 1:29). Fruits and vegetables were all that was deemed necessary for sustenance in the garden of Eden. However, much of the nutritional substances in these foods are concentrated in their natural raw juices. These juices are "locked up," you might say, in the cellulose fibers of the plant. In order to extract the nutrients, the body must break down the fibrous cells. This is a major chore for some digestive systems, particularly for the elderly, whose problems may be further complicated by faulty teeth or dentures that make it difficult to properly chew fibrous foods. Solid food requires many hours of digestive activity before its nourishment is finally available to the cells and tissues of the body. Juices, on the other hand, are quickly digested and assimilated, sometimes in a matter of a few minutes.

Juicing promises better health . . . . . .

In the interest of better health through easier digestion and assimilation, nutrition authorities like Norman Walker, Walther Schoenenberger and Paavo Airola recommend separating the juices from the fibrous materials before consuming them. This way, much of the nutritional benefit of a large amount of fruit or vegetable may be obtained simply by drinking a glass of juice. We can, of course, drink far more juice than we can comfortably

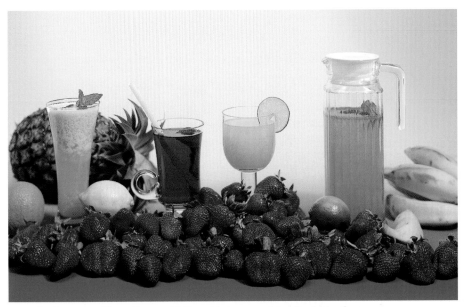

eat whole vegetables. About 2 kilos (4.4 pounds) of whole fruit or vegetable will make ½ - 1 liter (1 quart) of juice. Naturally, the juice has a higher concentration of minerals, vitamins, trace element, enzymes and valuable building materials for strong, healthy cells. Juice therapy—that is, drinking freshly extracted juices daily—will revitalize the body in an amazingly short time. Those with a poor appetite can drink their nourishment without having to force food into an unwilling stomach.

Those who suffer from stomach or intestinal ulcers often cannot eat raw vegetables, but they can easily drink soothing and healing carrot juice. Raw potato juice will do wonders for an ailing stomach. The juice is alkaline and will provide enzymes to aid digestion. But make no mistake: raw juices are not just for the sick and the ailing.

Raw juices are for everybody. As a matter of fact, nutritionally, juice therapy is the healthiest thing you can do for your body. Besides the water in the juice, which is pure and unadulterated, you receive minerals and vitamins, enzymes and trace element, all in their most natural, concentrated form. And unlike cooked food, the nutrients found in juices retain their natural molecule structure, which the body recognizes instantly and puts to work immediately—without a lengthy digestion time.

You are ingesting live food, that's why you feel better. I guarantee it, no matter what your state of health.

Start early . . . .

Raw carrot juice is excellent for babies. It can be mixed with milk and fed as soon as the baby needs a little more than just

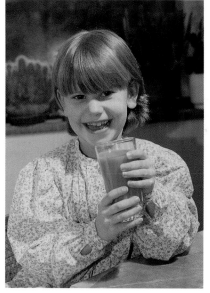

mother's milk. Straight carrot juice can be fed to babies after they are weaned; it provides the pro-vitamin beta-carotene as well as minerals, and contributes to rich blood and good skin color. There will be no colic, cradle cap or skin rashes–reactions often seen in babies given formula. And fresh carrot juice continues to be invaluable for growing children, who will drink the naturally sweet juice when it is sometimes impossible to coax them to eat their vegetables. For adolescents, carrot juice aids the normal development of glands and prevents, or helps to overcome, acne.

Above all, raw vegetable and fruit juices taken daily guarantee that the body receives its quota of building material for its trillions of cells. The daily dose of enzymes alone, which are not available from hamburgers or other cooked foods (because enzymes do not survive heat above 118° F or 48° C), will make a difference in how you feel. Think of enzymes as the catalyst–or the spark plugs–for a well functioning metabolism.

Without enzymes there is no digestion. It is true that the body produces most enzymes on its own, but as we grow older our bodies make less and less digestive enzymes. As we slow down, so too does our digestion. Lack of enzymes causes poor digestion, which in turn makes it difficult for the body to absorb nutrients from food intake. In the long run, the immune system weakens and we become more susceptible to sickness and disease. It is important, therefore, that we supply our bodies with more enzymes from raw juices. It's like making deposits in your own health bank account: If you keep on drawing cheques, that is using enzymes from the body's store without depositing fresh ones daily from food sources, one of these days your cheque will bounce. We see this demonstrated only too graphically in the case of the pancreas when it is over-burdened with refined carbohydrates. It finally gets tired and stops producing insulin. As a result diabetes sets in. Far too many middle-aged people (1 percent of the population) contract this disease every year, owing to an excessive intake of refined carbohydrates, white sugar and white flour in baking, pasta and processed, packaged foods.

Get energized . . . .

I must admit that I have not always followed the regime of daily fresh-pressed juices. I believed that being a vegetarian and eating fresh salads and raw foods daily, and otherwise adhering to a healthy whole foods diet (with the occasional glass of fresh juice thrown in) would keep me healthy.

And, indeed, I have not seen much sickness during my entire life, and the times I had to stay home because of the flu or cold I can probably count on my fingers. But as the years advanced and I came closer to retirement age, I experienced a lack of energy, and it started to bother me. I felt sluggish far too often. First I thought I needed to take longer vacations to revitalize. I took up gardening as a hobby and rented two large garden plots. I got my exercise digging, raking and weeding. It felt good to spend more time outdoors. But still something was missing. Then my wife, Christel, and I bought a new juicer, one that was able to make large quantities on a continuous basis. We started a regular routine of drinking a tall glass of freshly extracted juice every morning, and often for lunch as well. Our garden supplied plenty of

Fresh juices taste much better than bottled. And it is not only the flavor that is superior; fresh juices are nutritionally superior as well. What is really wrong with commercial juices is that they have all gone through a heat process that kills the all-important enzymes.

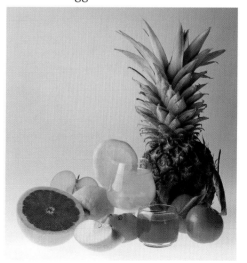

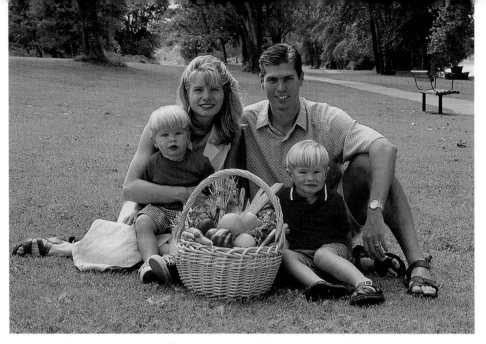

Organic vegetables–from your own garden or from an organic produce supplier–result in wonderfully nutritious juices.

organically-grown vegetables–carrots, red beets, lettuce, radishes, cucumbers, tomatoes and potatoes, watercress, garlic and onions, as well as several varieties of cabbage.

It is amazing the changes we have noticed! Now we feel energized and healthy and get through the day in high spirits. Visitors to our house have little choice, as they are invited to join in a tall glass of fresh juice. They also love it.

It is easy to share my enthusiasm for juicing with friends, relatives and colleagues. Few, however, adopt this habit. It seems to me that people will only change their lifestyle when disease or disaster strikes, when something goes wrong, when the doctors diagnose cancer, diabetes or heart disease. Why is it that people think juicing takes too much time? In reality it takes less time than it does to prepare breakfast and brew coffee. And if you eat out regularly you spend far more time traveling to and fro and waiting to be served than you would preparing freshly extracted juice at home. I guess it all boils down, so to speak, to

Juices provide tremendous support for the metabolic process, helping to eliminate toxins from the body and increase circulation, thereby strengthening the immune system immensely. Fresh juices contain easy-to-digest carbohydrates, fruit acids, pectins, phyto-hormones, enzymes, plenty of vitamins and minerals, as well as many vital and trace elements–they are a veritable fountain of youth.

how we plan and organize our time and ourselves. When we are sick in bed or in the hospital we are spending a lot more time getting healthy than we would have spent staying healthy. As the saying goes: The first part of our life we spend our time and health to get wealthy, while the second part of our life we spend our time and wealth to get healthy.

Fresh-pressed juices are alkaline. They purge the body of toxins by activating a cleansing of all cell structures, and by neutralizing excessive acids and creating an alkaline-acid balance. The metabolic process is constantly producing acids, especially with a carnivorous diet. The lack of a proper alkaline counter balance will inevitably lead to an overly acidic body environment, making the body susceptible to all kinds of ailments. An acidic body attracts colds and flu, rheumatoid arthritis and even cancer.

Juicing promises a long life . . . .

Taking care of your own body should be your greatest priority if you expect a long and healthy life. I encourage you to get into the habit of juicing on a daily basis. The benefits that go along with it are such that you will never want to give it up.

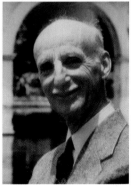

We would do well to follow the example of Norman Walker (1875-1985), the man responsible for popularizing juicing in the USA and Canada. This English-born businessman, who lived for 109 years, discovered the value of vegetable juices while recovering from a breakdown in a peasant house in the French countryside. While watching the women in the kitchen peel carrots, he noticed the moistness under the peel. He decided to try grinding them, and had his first cup of carrot juice!

When he recovered, Walker moved to Long Beach, California. Along with a medical doctor, he opened a juice bar and offered home delivery. From 1910 to 1930, they concocted dozens of fresh juice formulas for specific conditions. These recipes are now in the public domain, and are reflected in some of the formulas in the recipe section of this book.

Walker designed his own juicer in two parts: a grinder to

Fresh juice advocate Norman Walker lived to be 109. Walker believed that consuming fresh juice was the key to a healthy colon and thus to good health.

grind the vegetable or fruit, and a press to extract the juice. It was a machine designed for commercial operations, capable of pressing great quantities of juice. But when the San Francisco health department banned the sale of unpasteurized vegetable juices, Walker simplified the juicer and offered it for sale to the public, who were then able to press their own juice at home. This juicer is still available today, but because of its prohibitively high price of over CAN $3,000 it is seldom used for household purposes.

Buying a good juicer . . . .

Soon after we married, Christel and I invested in a small centrifugal juicer, which we used on and off. For example, we made

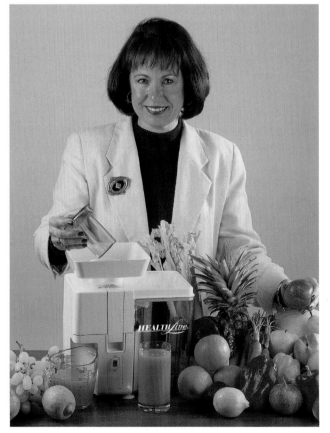

apple juice when apples were in season. Then as the family grew we began juicing carrots for the kids. They loved juice, especially in the morning for breakfast. I remember friends and other people remarking that all our kids had such healthy skin. It was the beta-carotene showing through.

Since the publication of my book *Healing with Herbal Juices* in 1993, I have received many letters and telephone calls from readers inquiring about the best machine for juicing the herbs described in the book. For that reason I added an extensive chapter on juicers to the second edition of that book. Here I will describe only the basic models and their functions. If you do not already have a juice extractor, I recommend you spend some time investigating the various models in order to determine what would best suit your lifestyle and pocket book.

Expeller-Press Juicers · · · · · · · · · · · ·

My first juicer was a little hand-cranked expeller-press juicer imported from Poland. It looks like an old-fashioned meat grinder with a long narrow spout and an adjustable screw to increase resistance and pressure. It does a wonderful job of extracting juice from practically anything–soft and hard fruit, berries, leafy vegetables as well as roots. One major drawback is that it is extremely time consuming and very tiring to press large amounts of fruit or vegetable juice. Most people buy this juicer for pressing small amounts of wheatgrass or herbal juice. The cost is around CAN $100.

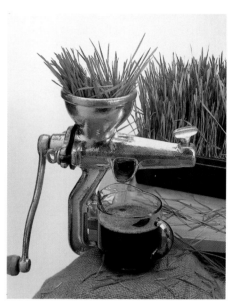

Electric Centrifugal Juicers · · · · · · · · ·

These are the juicers sold everywhere today. They come in either pulp-ejecting or non-pulp-ejecting models. As I mentioned earlier, it was a simple non-pulp-ejecting centrifugal juicer that Christel and I bought soon after we got married. These juicers are relatively inexpensive and they tend to be chosen by people who have never used a juicer before. The retail price is usually less than CAN $100, unless you purchase one of the top-of-the-line models, which cost around CAN $400. We had our small, inexpensive juicer for many years, but did not use it regularly as it didn't produce enough juice in one sitting for a growing family.

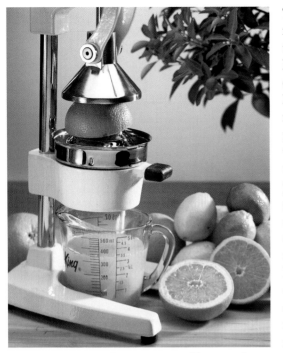

The pulp needed to be removed several times during the juicing process. If we had known how great the benefits of fresh juices really were, and how easy and quick it is to make plenty of juice with a pulp-ejecting model, we would have purchased one like that in the first place. Our old juicer finally ended up at a garage sale, and we invested in a good pulp-ejecting juice extractor. Not only was this new juicer fun to use (even the kids loved to make juice) it was easy to operate and quick to clean. We made delicious juices from apples, pears and other fruit, and vegetable cocktails using carrots, red beets, celery, tomatoes, potatoes, radish, as well as many different combinations, which you will find in the recipe section.

The pulp-ejector type juicer is the most popular juicer sold today. They come in many different models and in all price ranges, some selling at mass merchandisers for as little as US $40 or CAN $60, and others as high as US $300 or CAN $450. But let me caution you: it is unwise to even consider purchasing an inexpensive centrifugal pulp-ejecting juicer for less than US $100 or CAN $145. The cheaper models all have a small and weak motor that is not built for daily juicing or for pressing large quantities of juice at a time. The most common complaint is that the weak motor is easily strained and burns out quickly, often shortly after the six-month warranty runs out.

On the other hand, you don't necessarily need to purchase the most expensive model either. For between around US $150.00 or CAN $225.00 you should be able to get a quality-built, reliable pulp-ejecting juice extractor with a strong motor and at least a three-year warrantee. It is also important that the cutting blade is made of surgical steel, and that the strainer or sieve is not made of aluminum, as they are in most cheap models. I have seen juicers with aluminum sieves where the fruit acid over time has chewed out big holes. Of course the aluminum ends up in the juice you drink, and we now know about the connection between aluminum overload and Alzheimer's. So, be aware, and look for quality rather than price. The Health-Line juicer is one model I really like; it fits the bill, is reliable, can handle an extended period of juicing and is an all-round quality machine. Nutrition stores and health and fitness centers usually carry quality brand names and give excellent service.

Masticating Juicers . . . .

These juicers are in a class of their own, not only price-wise but also in how they work. The two most popular ones are the *Champion* and the *GreenLife*.

The Champion was introduced in the late 1950s. It has a rotating cutter on a shaft made of stainless steel. It first grates, then masticates or chews the pulp to further break down the cell wall structure, and then mechanically squeezes and presses the pulp through a narrowing spout to extract the juice. The pulp is automatically ejected.

Almost every type of vegetable, even leafy ones, can be juiced with the Champion. The fruit juice, however, is a bit on the pulpy side, bordering on fruit sauce. Since its introduction, the Champion has not undergone any significant structural changes or

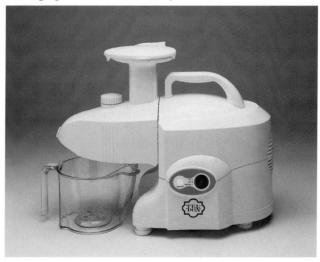

improvements. The cost has remained stable at about US $295 or CAN $450.

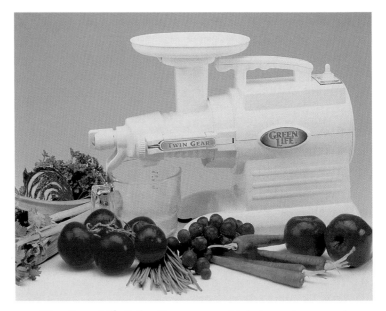

The GreenLife Juice Extractor, which is an improved, yet lower-priced, version of the more sophisticated GreenPower juicer from Korea, represents the highest advancement in juicing technology in quite a long time. What sets the GreenLife apart is that it can juice just about anything: hard fruits and vegetables, soft fruits like pineapple and berries, celery sticks, all types of herbs without exception, sprouts and even wheatgrass. It slowly and carefully crushes and presses fruits and vegetables as well as leafy greens using a unique twin-gear triturating extraction system (a combination of grinding, pressing and pushing through) that operates at a very low speed of only 90 rpm.

Another excellent and revolutionary feature found only in the GreenLife, and of course in its forerunner the GreenPower juicer, are the magnetic rollers, which, while pressing the juice out, magnetize the juice and so delay the start of oxidation. This feature alone, which is not offered by any other juicer, is sure to justify the price of US $595 or CAN $795 for the sophisticated juicer enthusiast. The GreenLife represents the cutting edge in juicer technology. It has won several prizes and medals at international exhibitions.

Therapeutic uses of vegetable juice . . .

You don't have to be sick to benefit from drinking raw juices. Think of it simply as your own health insurance plan. Many people take vitamin and mineral supplements, or are on some sort of program that might include one of the many green powders or dried juice mixtures. These supplements have been researched by Dr. Yoshihide Hagiwara, and have recently become very popular owing to their promotion by Sam Gracie, Harvey Diamond and multi-level sales organizations. Incorporating these food supplements into the daily routine is certainly an excellent idea; again, it's like investing in a good health insurance policy. But there is a better policy: drinking fresh juices, which are a much superior source of natural vitamins, minerals and enzymes than those that are man-made in a laboratory. I am not saying that if you are taking the green powders you should discontinue them. On the contrary, when added to fresh-pressed juices you get a double whammy of nutrients, including enzymes and the life element.

The fact is that none of the supplements supply the life element that is present in freshly pressed raw juices. And keep in mind that all nutrients influence each other by working synergistically; that is, they help each other to create reactions within the body—just like clockwork, where each little wheel depends on the other. Only fresh juices provide these perfect conditions.

What is this "life element," exactly? . . .

Dr. Werner Kollath (1892 - 1970)

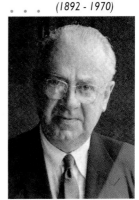

The life element is not a substance, and science has not been able to isolate it or preserve it. Dr. Werner Kollath (1892-1970), a physician, hygienist and nutritional scientist in Germany, along with Dr. Herbert Shelton (1895-1985) and Dr. Norman Walker (1876-1985) were the first on this continent to make significant advancements toward an understanding of the difference between living food and dead food. Kollath's nutritional advice was simple and direct: leave food as natural as possible. He proved scientifically that a per-

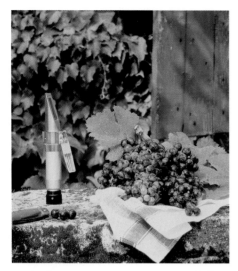

A refractometer measures the sugar content in grapes, wine and juice.

son could eat enough to seem healthy and still be suffering from malnutrition. To describe food of optimum quality, Kollath introduced the concept of "full value," meaning that the nutrients typically contained by a specific food are fully preserved in their natural form—that is, raw and uncooked. The life element is contained in grain, which is why it sprouts when the conditions are right. Any food that is irradiated will not sprout any longer because the enzymes have been killed and the life element destroyed. The food is dead and will start to decompose as soon as it is exposed to oxygen. Don't be fooled by all the publicity fuelled by commercial interest that would have us believe that the process of irradiation preserves food. It preserves it only as an inert, dead element. Microwaving, too, has the same deadly effect.

When food is cooked not only does it lose the action of the enzymes, which are destroyed by heat, it also loses its natural nutritional value. Protein (especially milk protein), for example, is altered; after cooking it is much harder to digest. During cooking all minerals go through a change of molecule structure and many vitamins are lost. You will, of course, get some benefits from cooked foods, as long as there are still enzymes present to make the nutrients available to the body. However, the elderly suffer from a lack of digestive enzymes, resulting in a slower rate of metabolism, which in turn speeds up the aging process.

If we look at the average person's diet today—which consists mostly of cooked, processed and refined foods, including preservatives, chemical additives and artificially-hardened fats—is it any wonder that there is a steady increase in heart disease, arteriosclerosis, high blood pressure, cancer and the breaking down of the immune system with all its consequences?

Choose complete living food

I have a hard time sharing the thinking and philosophy of modern science, both in the pharmaceutical and the nutritional arenas. These researchers and scientists are actually doing something that is, from the whole- and life-foods perspective, really silly. They are constantly isolating nutrients, looking for active ingredients, then, when they have isolated them, they put them back together again, marketing them as neutraceuticals or "designer" foods. It is like cutting up a living dog, studying the different parts, selecting the superior ones, putting them all together again and then honestly expecting that these isolated parts will create a "super" dog. Too bad for my scientist friends, but the dog is dead and will decompose in time.

Life and health can be sustained only with complete living food. When the life element is missing from our food we will without doubt degenerate also.

Fighting Cancer

There is scientific proof of cancer-fighting properties in fresh juices. Almost everything we know about the health benefits of drinking fresh juices has come to us through empirical evidence. What that means is that we have gained insight and learned by observation and experience, contrary to learning from clinical studies that require a minimum of 36 people in a

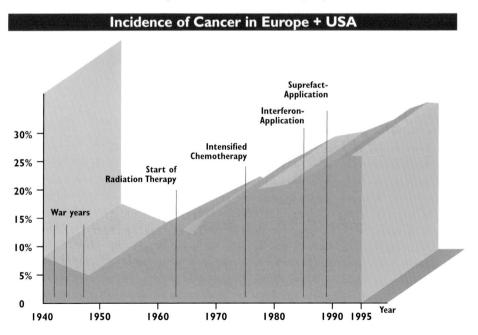

Incidence of Cancer in Europe + USA

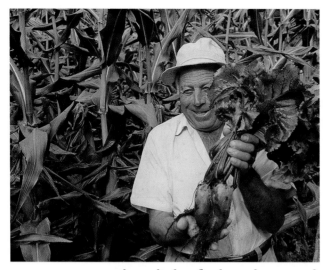

double-blind study. (Eighteen of the participants are being administered the real thing while the others are given a placebo.) Clinical studies usually require the participation of three doctors. That is why clinical studies cost a minimum of $450,000 dollars. Because of this enormous cost, double-blind studies are rarely applied to food supplement or herbal medicine research, as neither product can be patented, and thus there is no great financial gain.

Nevertheless, scientists have recently looked into the health effects of certain food substances and learned that cruciferous vegetables (those from the entire cabbage family), as well as tomatoes, spinach and carrots, contain important cancer inhibitors known as lycopene and alpha- and beta-carotenes. *The European Journal of Nutrition* (issue 38, 1999), reports on a study conducted by researcher Dr. H. Müller, et al. In this study, twenty-three males were given a daily glass of fresh lycopene-rich tomato juice and an alpha- and beta-carotene-rich carrot juice together with 10 grams of lutein-rich spinach powder. The results showed a significant improvement of carotene concentration in the blood. The scientists concluded that a daily intake of fresh juice guarantees the cells an abundant supply of oxygen.

It is a well-known fact that a lack of oxygen on a cell level triggers the beginning of the cancer tumor. Dr. Otto Warburg discovered this phenomenon in the 1930s, for which he received the Nobel Prize. He is the only medical doctor to receive an unshared Nobel Prize for medicine not only once but twice, and basically for the same discovery: namely, that a lack of oxygen causes cancer. Now we have scientific proof to add to the empirical evidence.

Juice Therapy

There are a number of famous doctors and practioners who use juice therapy as a part of their treatment programs. Dr. Anne Wigmore of the original Hippocrates Institute in Baltimore used mainly fresh wheatgrass juice for her cancer patients. Her teachings found followers worldwide. The Hungarian physician and scientist Alexander Ferenczi had great success with red beet juice. In the 1950s Ferenczi observed that a colleague had successfully used red beet root juice in the treatment of leukemia patients. Encouraged by these results, Ferenczi conducted a study with a group of twenty-two patients, all with advanced, inoperable cancers. They all received 30 milliliters of fresh red beet juice daily. After three months, twenty-one patients showed marked improvements. He observed that the red beet therapy was a natural remedy of apparent efficacy without any side effects. In addition, this treatment was inexpensive and available in unlimited quantity.

Positive results are also achieved at the Gerson Institute in Mexico under the direction of Charlotte Gerson. She still uses the raw juice formulas created by her father, the famous German doctor Max Gerson. Though very successful in his practice of using fresh juices, he was persecuted in the United States, accused of "unprofessional conduct" for treating the very sick

Fresh vegetable and fruit juices are the best source of antioxidants– there is no doubt about it.

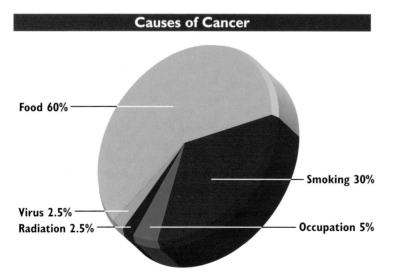

Causes of Cancer

Food 60%

Smoking 30%

Virus 2.5%
Radiation 2.5%

Occupation 5%

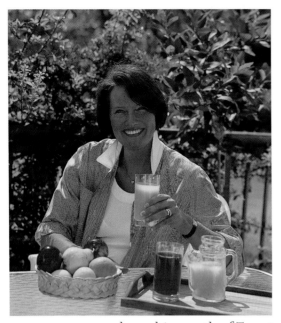

and those with terminal cancer. He had to relocate to Mexico.

Most recently Dr. George Malkmus has attracted much attention with his "Hallelujah" healing diet, which includes drinking fresh juices daily. Having healed himself from colon cancer with raw juices and a diet he discovered on the first pages of the bible, he decided to teach his raw juice therapy to thousands of health ministers in his seminars at Hallelujah Acres located in North Carolina, and at a Canadian branch in Ontario, about an hour drive north of Toronto. It is overwhelming to see the healings and changes for the better in all kinds of people suffering from degenerative diseases.

To cite just one more report–this by the research scientist Dr. A. Nagoyva, and published in the *Annals of Nutrition and Metabolism* (issue 42, 1998). Four Slovenian scientists observed nineteen lacto-ovo vegetarians and their controlled intake of antioxidants with their food. The results showed that antioxidants in sufficient quantities prevent arteriosclerosis (plugged-up arteries). Fresh vegetable and fruit juices are the best source of antioxidants–there is no doubt about it.

So, if you are worried about plugged-up arteries, which usually first show with a warning sign of elevated blood pressure, take my advice and get into the habit of drinking fresh juices daily. Recent studies link heart disease, high blood pressure, cancer, arthritis and many other degenerative diseases to an overload of animal protein in our diets. Research concerning the link between excess animal protein and disease has shown the elimination of animal meat to be absolutely essential in the prevention and treatment of cancer. A shift to a plant-based diet with plenty of fresh juices results not only in significant improvements in health but often in total cures.

Some people get really nervous when they hear the word "fasting." "How can I survive without solid food?" they ask. Rest assured, to fast is not to starve. It is a positive thing to do. Fasting—not eating solid food for a period of time—is an ancient practice. We know through literature and biblical records that people fasted for long periods of time. Jesus fasted for forty days as recorded in the gospels. We can also read in Greek literature that in ancient days sick people abstained from food for up to fourteen days before being given plant extracts to facilitate healing and a speedy recovery. And isn't our first reflex to reduce food intake when we are not feeling well? A short juice fast of three or four days has proven to be an excellent way to rid the body of waste and toxins, thereby increasing energy and vitality. Those who have done a short juice fast for the first time often report having experienced their first glimpse of true well-being.

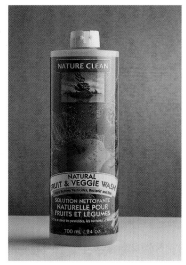

Nowadays it is easy to do a juice fast. Organic fruits and vegetables, my first choice, are usually readily available. And if I can't get organic produce I buy regular, fresh produce at the supermarket. I do, however, make sure that I clean it thoroughly, especially the fruit, as it is often sprayed for cosmetic reasons.

Every so often I hear people commenting that they cannot afford a daily organic cocktail due to the high cost of the vegetables. Frankly, I feel it is all a matter of perception. A weeks' supply of fresh produce can be less expensive than the price of a hair cut, a movie ticket or the cost of a meal at a restaurant. Paying now for *staying* healthy, in my view, is still a better choice than paying later for *becoming* healthy. As the saying goes, an ounce of prevention is better than a pound of cure.

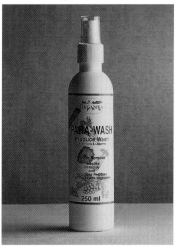

Non-toxic fruits and vegetables

Don't panic—use organic. For juicing I prefer organically grown fruits and vegetables.

Fortunately they are becoming widely available at reasonable prices also.

Sometimes it is impossible to get organics. In that case I make sure the fruits are carefully washed with a non-toxic fruit and vegetable wash which removes residues of pesticides and chemical sprays, as well as bacteria, e-coli and even salmonella, should that ever be present.

Let's get started . . . .

When you start juicing you will soon discover specific juices for which you will develop a liking. I myself prefer vegetables to fruit, while Christel, my wife, loves carrot juice best.

The following is a partial list of suitable ingredients for juices. Juicing is fun, or at least it should be. Experiment with different combinations of fruit. In general, I do not mix fruit and vegetables, however carrot and apple make a lovely juice. Try them all and surprise yourself.

Excellent Juicing Ingredients			
Fruits			
pineapple	grapefruit	melon	coconut
apricot	plums	cherries	quince
peach	prunes	grape	pomegranate
orange	papaya	rhubarb	
tangerine	apple	mango	
Vegetables			
asparagus	beet root	tomato	leek
carrots	red kale	peppers	pumpkin
cucumber	cabbage	turnip	borage
string beans	kohlrabi	Swiss chard	fennel
green beans	potato	broccoli	artichoke
Brussels sprouts	bean sprouts	lettuce	
cauliflower	Jerusalem	celery	
red radishes	artichoke	zucchini	
Spices			
onion	ginger	scallions	parsley
garlic			

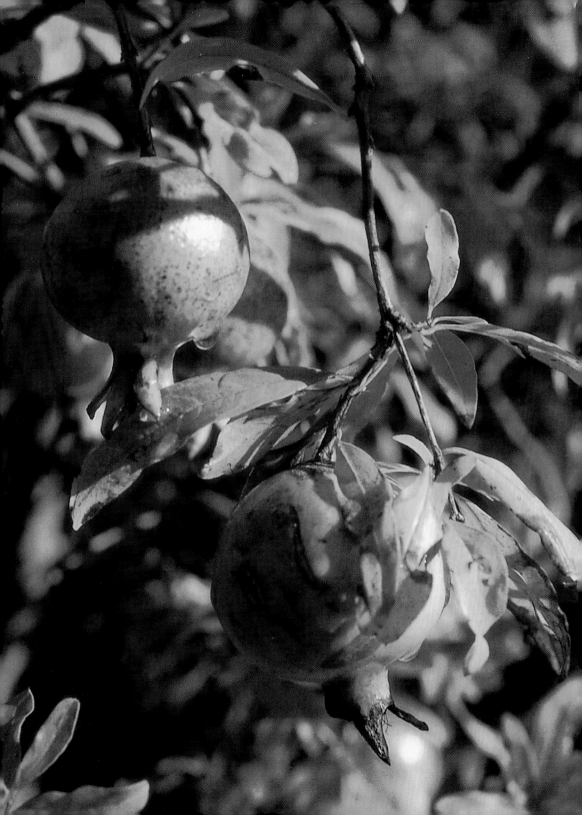

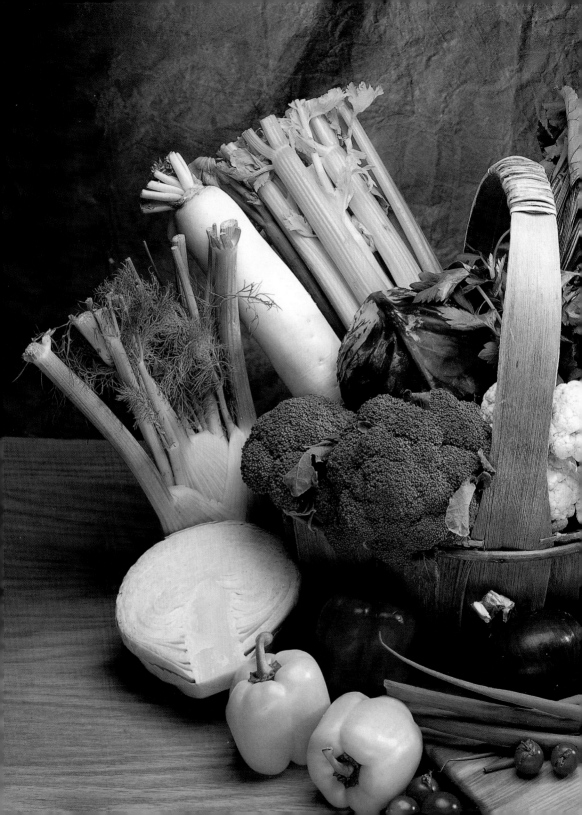

Juice Recipes

In the following section a combination of several different juices are recommended for the treatment of specific ailments. To simplify matters I have included the quantity for each of the ingredients. Frankly, I hardly ever stick to a recipe, but vary the recipes according to what I have available. If you run short or don't have some of the ingredients it really does not matter. Do without it for the time being. The quantity, therefore, signifies the parts recommended in the formula, a little more or less will do no harm.

Should you juice enough to last for several days? I would say no. Some say that juice, if stored in an airtight container and refrigerated, will last for several days. However, I find that day-old juice has not only lost its fresh taste, but has started to deteriorate because of the oxidizing process. It starts at a slow pace but gains momentum with time. You will certainly not lose all nutrients overnight, but you will lose some.

Acidic Stomach

heartburn

3 raw potatoes

3 carrots

I apple

I stalk celery

apple

potato

Acne

pimples, non-infectious blemishes

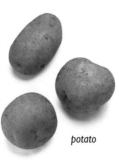

artichoke

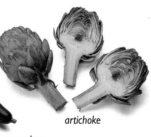

cucumber

4 carrots

I cucumber

I whole lemon (scrape off oily outer skin)

I raw potato

I artichoke

I apple

alternatively

2 apples

I bunch red grapes

6 apricots (when in season)

For best results prepare about ½ - 1 liter of juice in the morning. Drink equal parts of the juice three times a day. If you are taking the juice for specific ailments it is advisable to take these formulas therapeutically for at least three weeks. You may continue with the therapy as long as you wish, as there are no unpleasant side effects known to any of the formulas. Should you ever find the taste too strong for your palate, dilute the juice with equal parts of water.

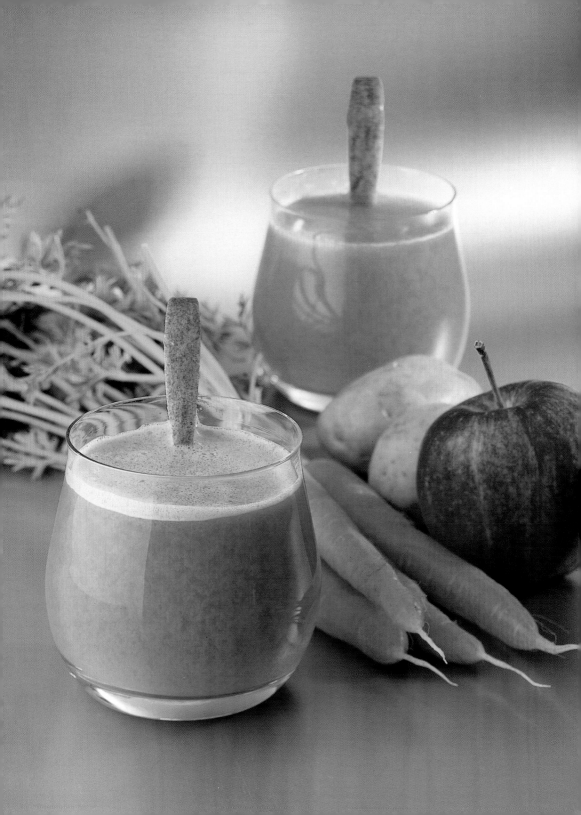

Anemia

Iron deficiency

4 carrots

1 red beet

1 celery stick

1 bunch spinach

1 bunch watercress

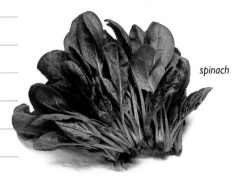

spinach

Angina Pectoris

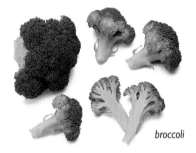

broccoli

6 carrots

1 red beet

1 bunch spinach

1 cucumber

2 green cabbage leaves,
kale or broccoli

Arteriosclerosis

8 carrots

1 clove garlic

1 red beet

2 stalks celery

garlic

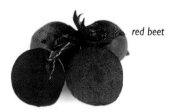

red beet

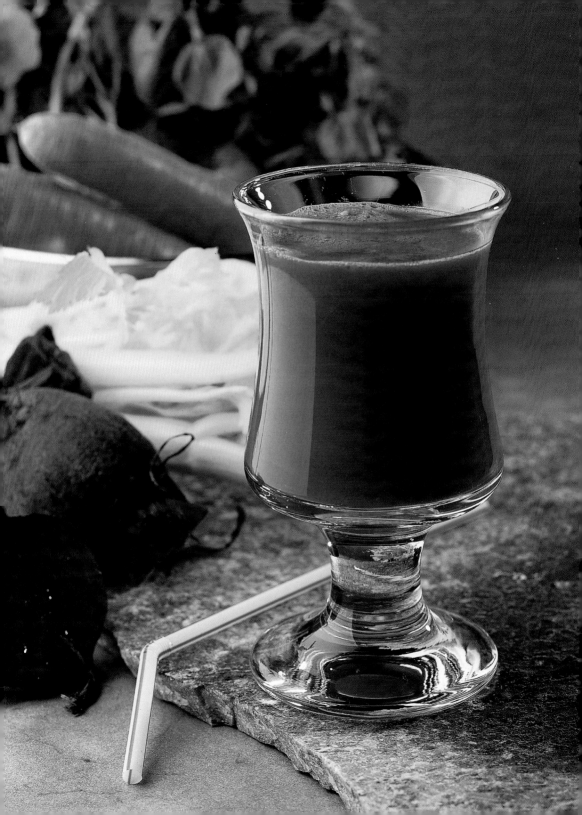

Arthritis

6 carrots

1 stalk celery

1 heaping tbsp fresh horseradish

1 cucumber

1 bunch spinach

alternatively

cherry juice, blueberry juice, blackberry juice
(Juice in season, freeze in freezer bags, drink one glass three times daily)

carrot

cucumber

Asthma

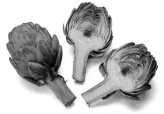

artichoke

red radish

6 carrots

1 artichoke

1 black radish or 6 red radishes

1 bunch spinach

1 stalk celery

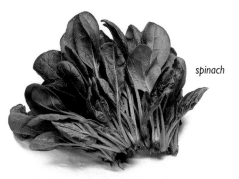

spinach

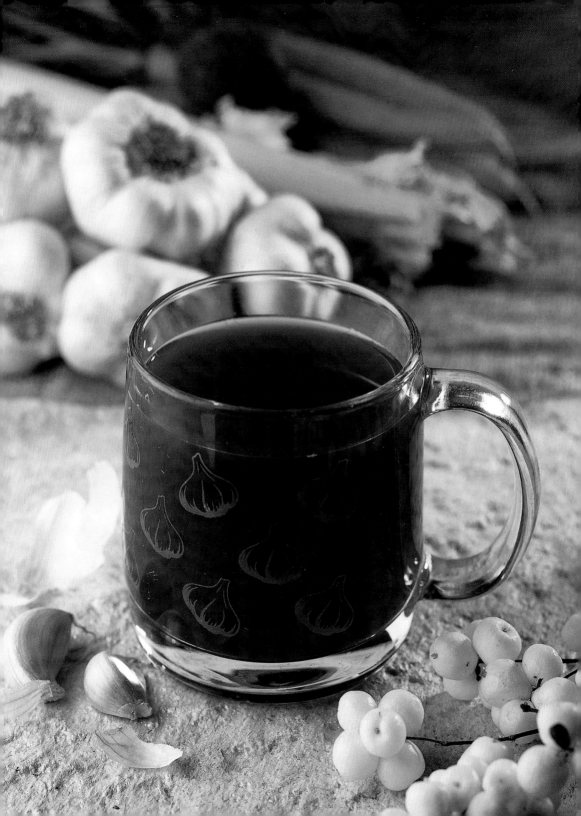

Bladder

cold or infection

6 carrots

1 green bell pepper

1 stalk celery

2 tomatoes

6 green and yellow leaves endive
(Belgium or curly)

alternatively

3 apples

1 cup cranberries
(fresh or frozen)

1 large slice watermelon

green bell pepper

tomato

cranberries

Blood Pressure

high

6 carrots

2 stalks celery

1 red beet

1 bunch parsley

1 clove garlic

1 bunch spinach

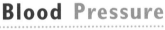

garlic

celery

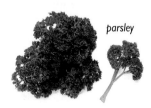

parsley

34

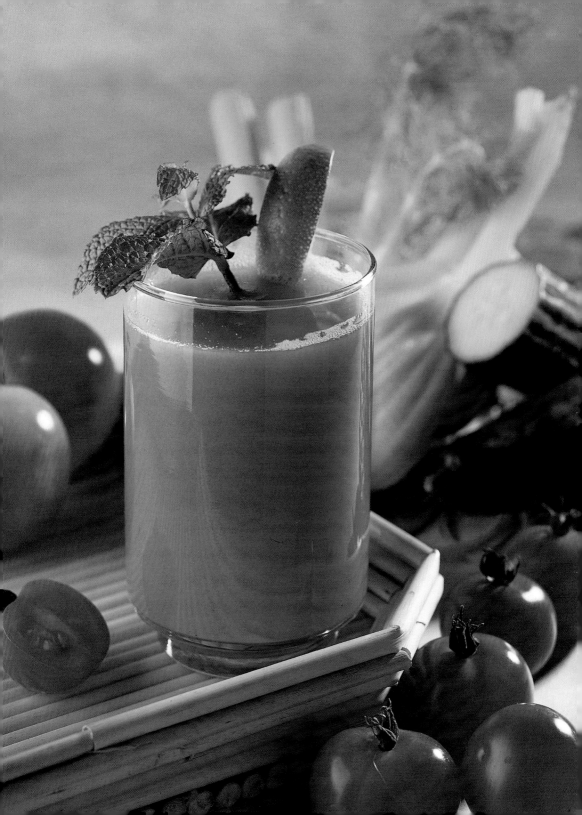

Bronchitis

4 carrots

¼ fennel root

1 tomato

1 cucumber

1 celery stalk

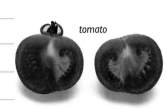

tomato

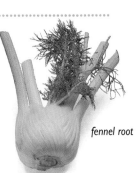

fennel root

Cancer

Red grapes, apples, lemons, carrots, red beets, celery, cruciferous vegetables (all members of the cabbage family), tomatoes, sunflower and clover sprouts, garden sorrel, as well as fresh (uncooked) sauerkraut juice are all very beneficial. The following cocktails will give you guidance as to what can be combined for a good tasting juice-and don't forget the garlic.

6 carrots

1 red beet

1 celery stalk

1 small bunch sorrel

2 cabbage leaves, cauliflower, broccoli or mustard leaves

1 clove garlic

alternatively

1 bunch of red grapes

2 apples

1 lemon, scrape away oily peel and juice whole lemon

lemon

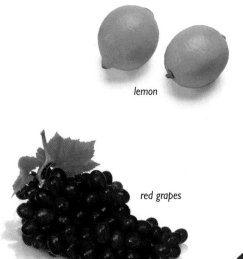

red grapes

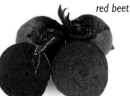

red beet

36

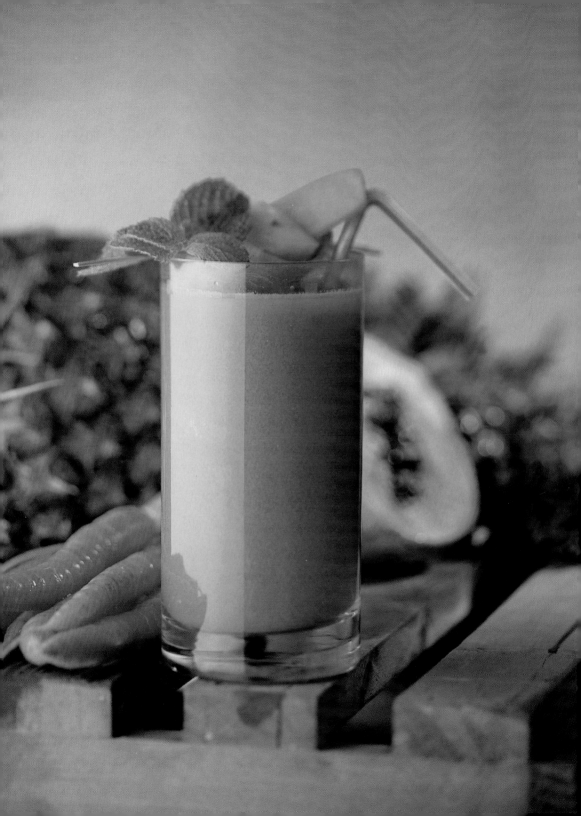

Candida

Yeast Infection

4 carrots

2 cabbage leaves

2 broccoli florets

4 radishes with green tops

1 clove garlic

alternatively

1 red beet

2 stalks celery

1 cucumber

1 bunch sunflower sprouts

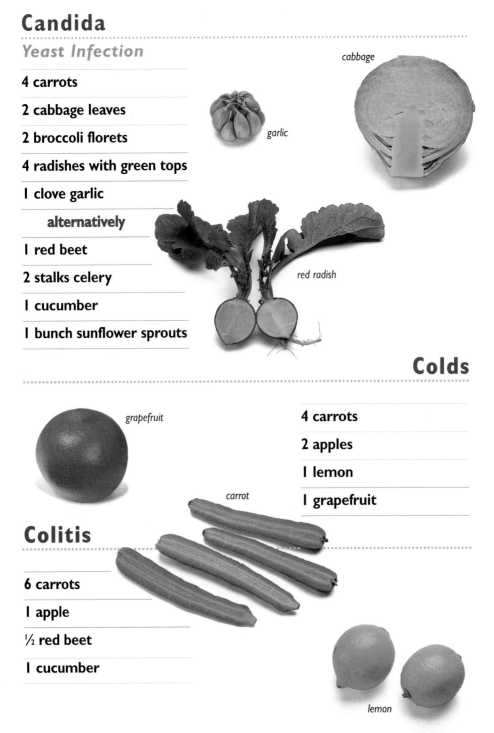

cabbage

garlic

red radish

Colds

4 carrots

2 apples

1 lemon

1 grapefruit

grapefruit

carrot

Colitis

6 carrots

1 apple

½ red beet

1 cucumber

lemon

38

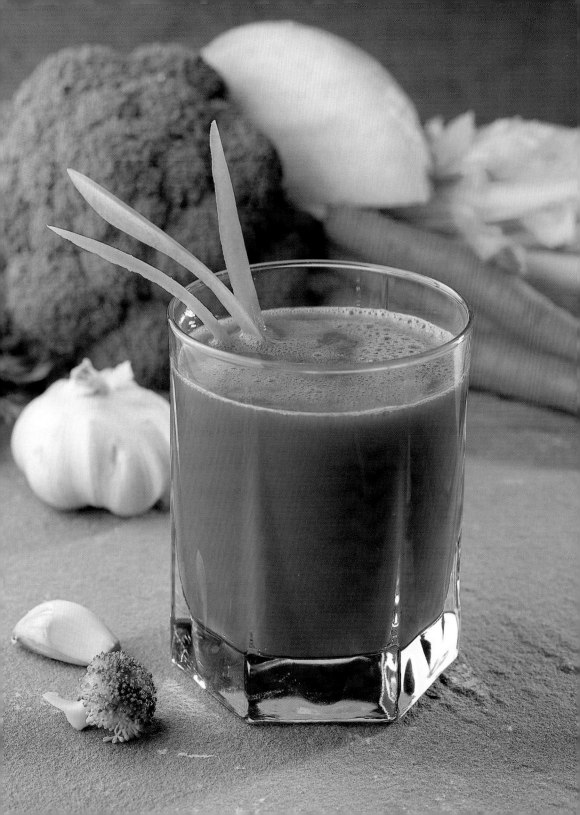

Constipation

4 carrots

I apple (Granny Smith)

I cup raw sauerkraut

alternatively

I cup raw sauerkraut

I apple (Granny Smith, Northern spy, McIntosh)

½ head butter or leaf lettuce

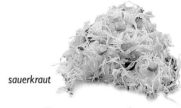

apple

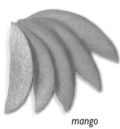

sauerkraut

Depression

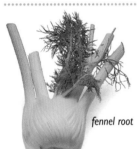

fennel root

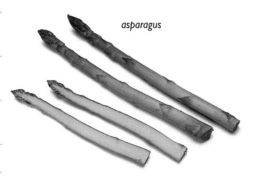

mango

I large bunch fresh borage herbs with flowers

I medium fennel root

I mango

Diabetes Mellitus

2 handfuls (5 cups) green string beans

3 roots Jerusalem artichoke

¼ medium size white or green cabbage

5 stalks asparagus

I cucumber

asparagus

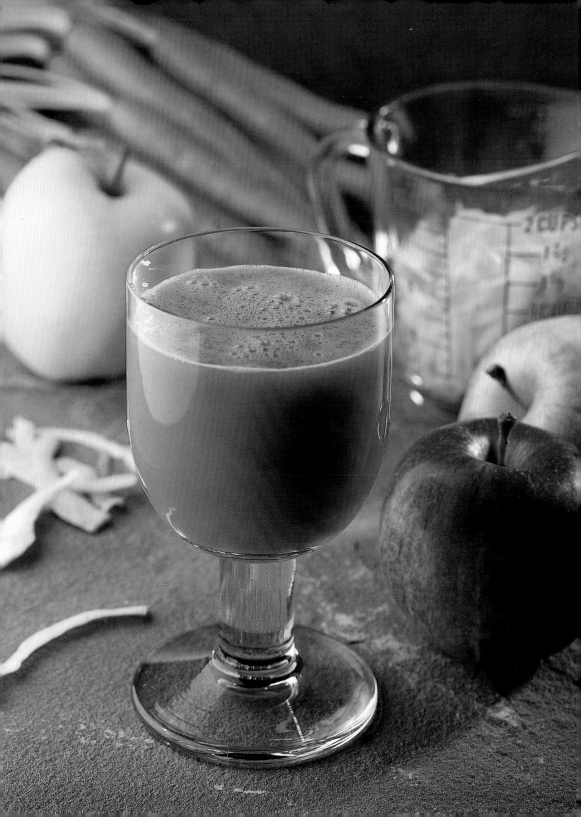

Diarrhea

4 carrots

1 apple

1 cup frozen blackberries

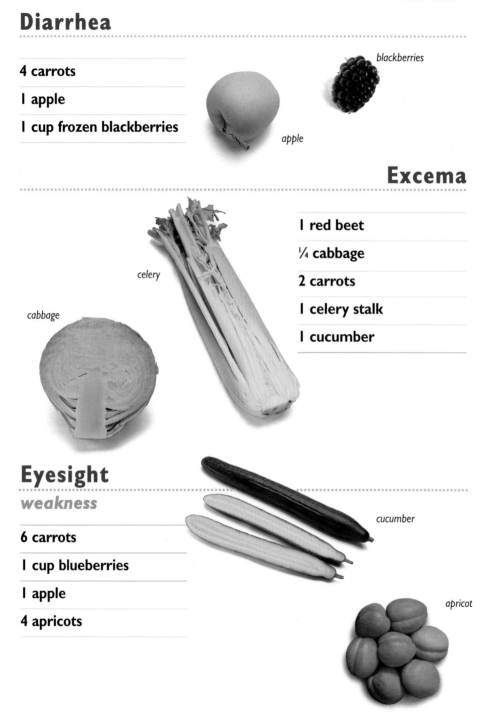

blackberries

apple

Excema

1 red beet

¼ cabbage

2 carrots

1 celery stalk

1 cucumber

celery

cabbage

Eyesight

weakness

6 carrots

1 cup blueberries

1 apple

4 apricots

cucumber

apricot

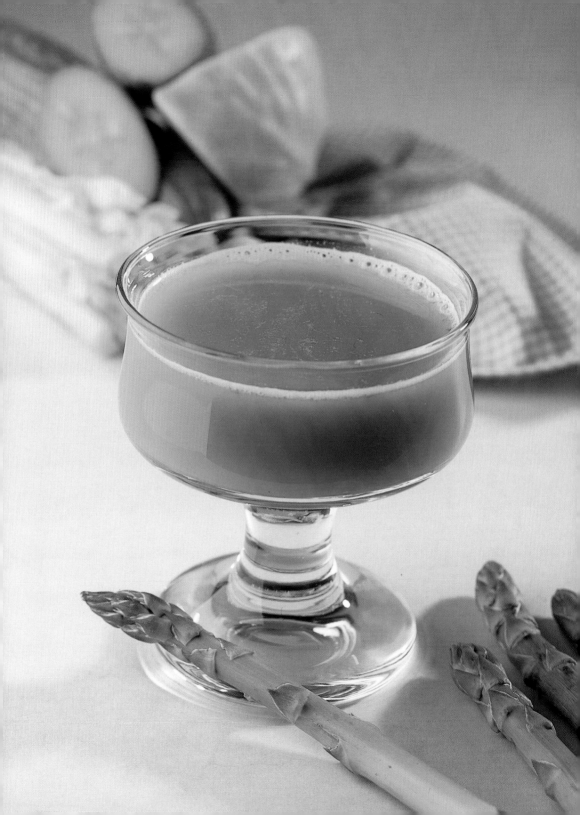

Fibromyalgia

5 carrots

¼ small turnip

I bunch watercress

I celery stalk

½ lemon

I clove garlic

lemon

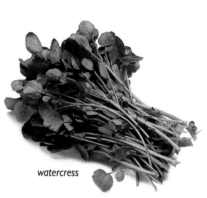

watercress

Gall Bladder Stones

inflammation

3 pears

3 round slices pineapple

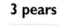

pear

44

Gall Bladder Cleanser

6 carrots

I small beet

½ lemon

6 red radishes or I black radish

black radish

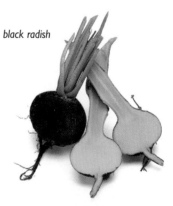

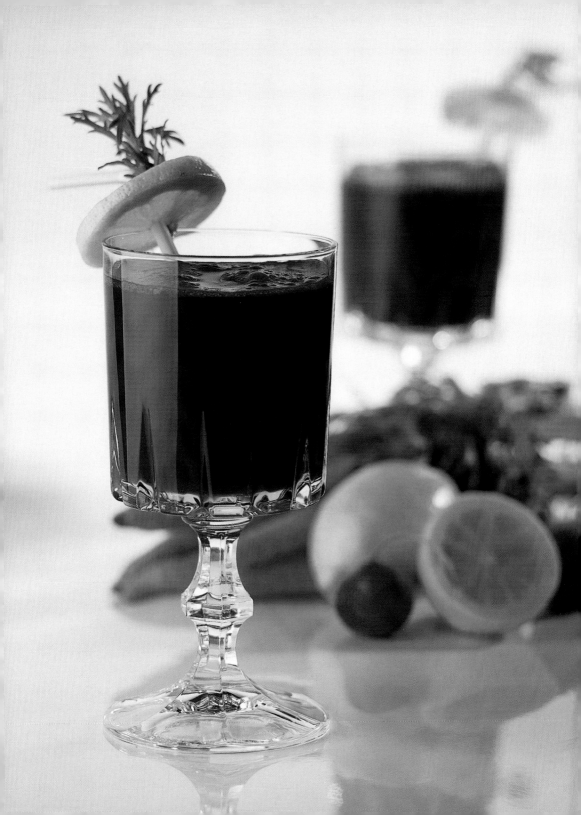

Gout

6 carrots

I celery stalk

I small red beet

I cucumber

I bunch watercress

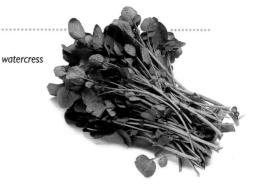

watercress

celery

Hypoglycemia

I small red beet

I celery stalk

6 red radishes or I black radish

6 large leaves green curly endive

Indigestion

papaya

2 carrots

I stalk celery

I raw potato

I thumb size fresh ginger root

¼ medium green cabbage

¼ fennel root

alternatively

I medium papaya, seeded

3 slices pineapple

potato

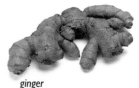

ginger

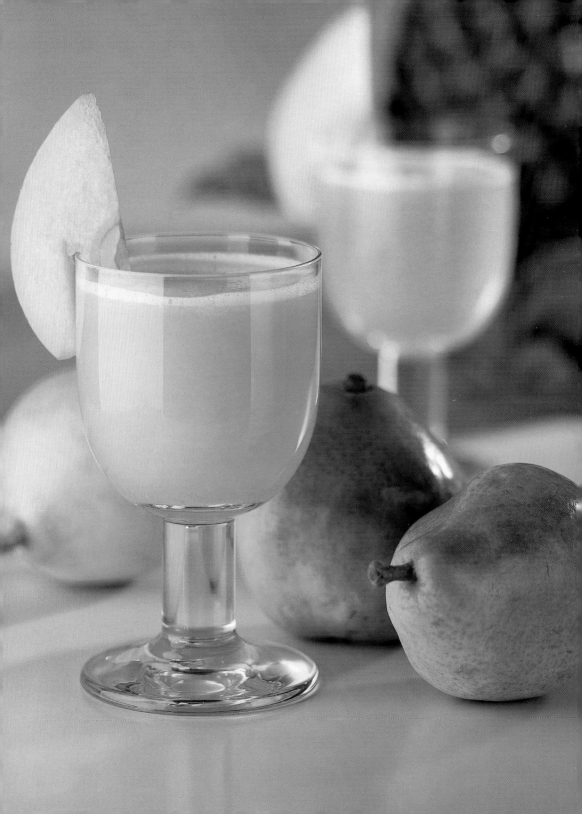

Influenza

Flu

6 carrots

2 celery stalks

**2 green leaves cabbage or
4 Brussels sprouts**

½ lemon

alternatively 1

6 tomatoes

4 radishes

1 bell pepper

1 celery stalk

½ lemon

1 thumb size ginger root

alternatively 2

1 large grapefruit

2 apples

½ lemon

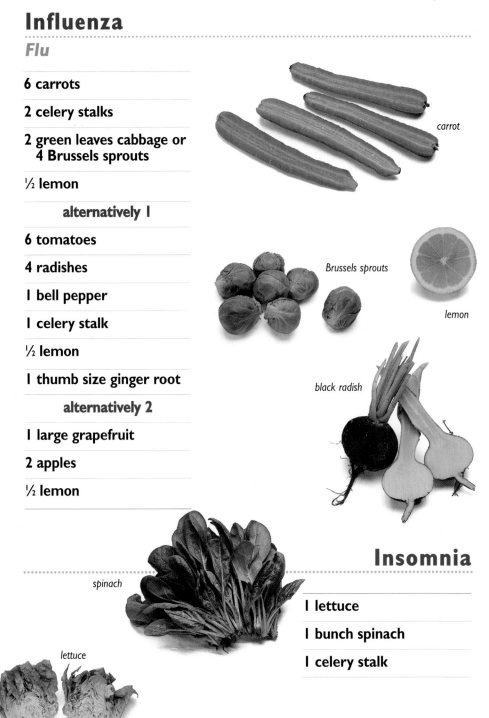

carrot

Brussels sprouts

lemon

black radish

spinach

Insomnia

1 lettuce

1 bunch spinach

1 celery stalk

lettuce

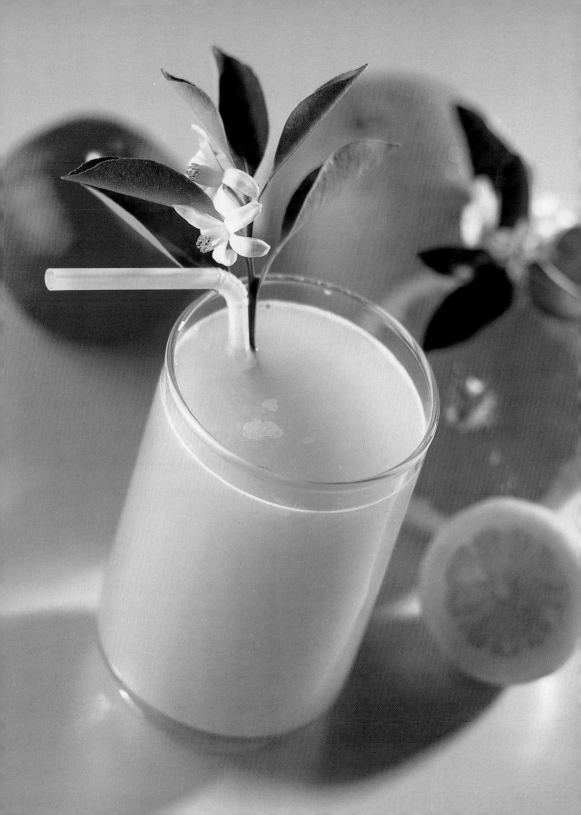

Kidney Trouble

3 celery stalks

2 tomatoes

I lemon, peeled

2 carrots

6 large green leaves
endive lettuce

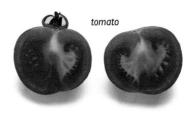
tomato

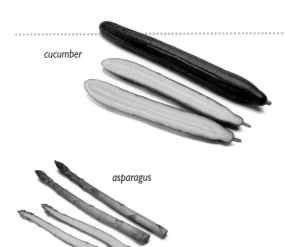
cucumber

asparagus

Liver Disorders

I Black radish or 6 - 8 red
radishes

12 large green and yellow
leaves curly endive

6 stalks asparagus

3 carrots

I cucumber

Mucus Membrane

dry

6 carrots

3 slices pineapple

½ papaya, seeded

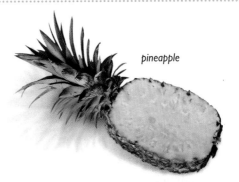
pineapple

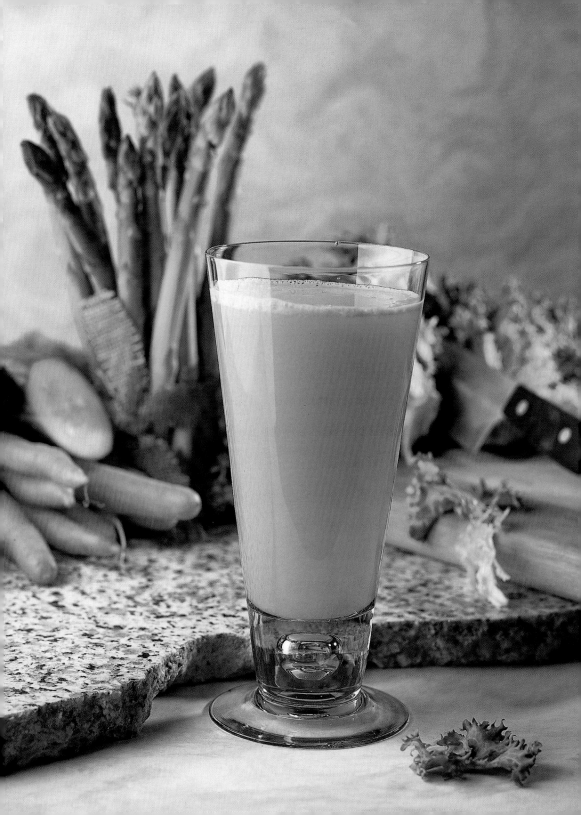

Nervousness

4 carrots

I celery stalk

I head butter lettuce

8 large green and yellow leaves curly

2 handful string beans

6 Brussels sprouts

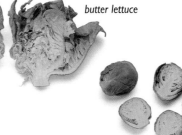

butter lettuce

Brussels sprouts

Osteoporosis

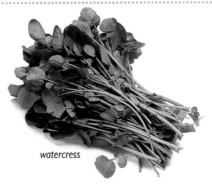

watercress

½ cabbage

I bell pepper

I cucumber

I bunch watercress

4 green leaves kale

Parasites

¼ cabbage

I black radish

I kilo (apx. 3 cups) pumpkin, cubed

I thumb-size ginger root

pumpkin

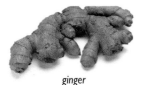

ginger

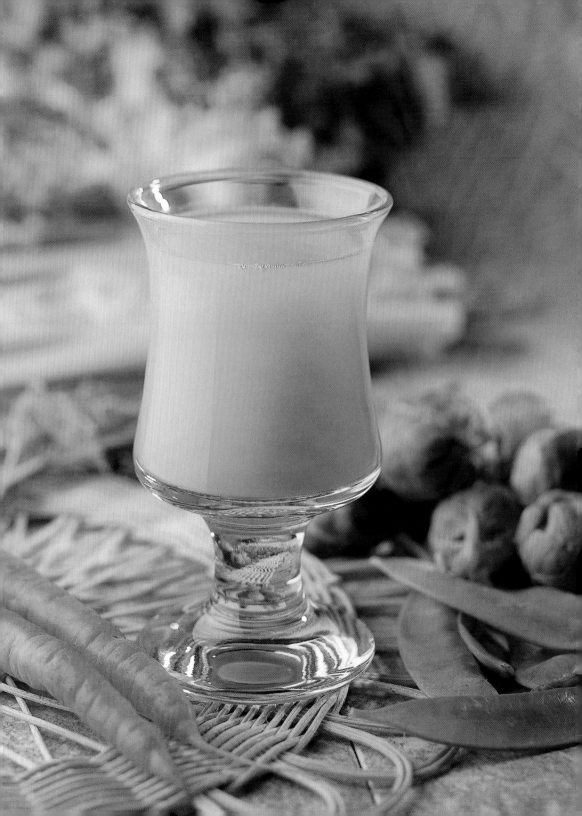

Peptic or Gastric Ulcers

¼ **green cabbage**

1 potato

2 celery stalks

6 carrots

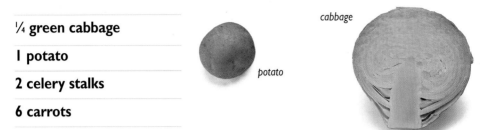

potato

cabbage

Prostate Problems

1 head butter lettuce

6 asparagus stalks

6 carrots

butter lettuce

asparagus

Psoriasis

5 carrots

1 cucumber

1 bunch spinach

1 celery stalk

spinach

carrot

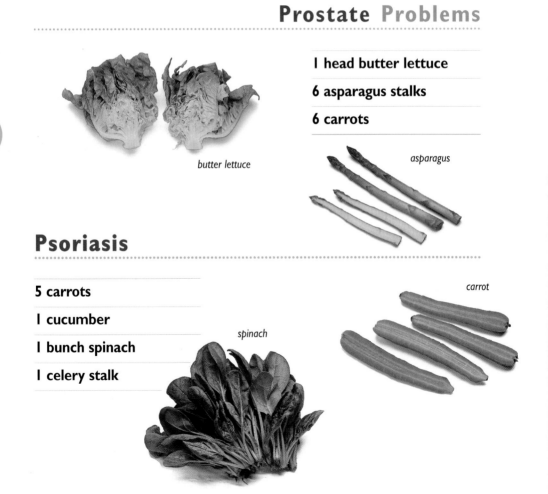

54

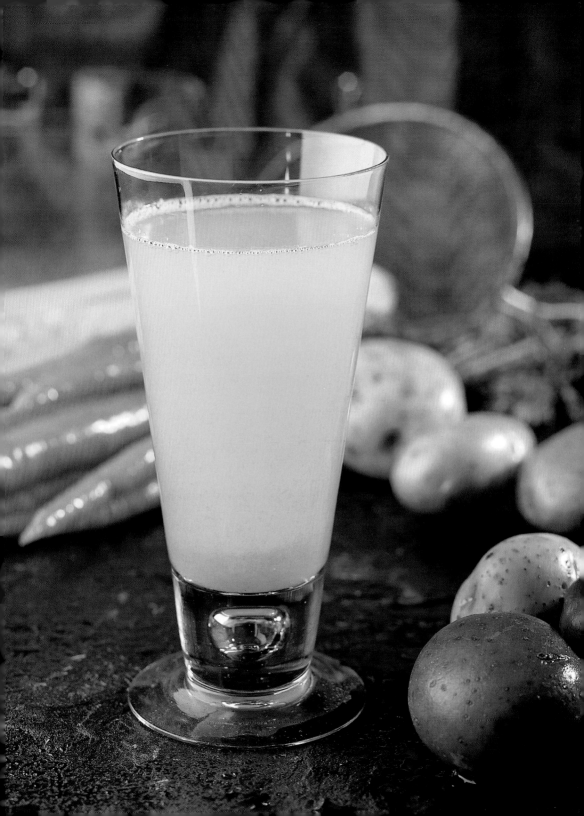

Rheumatism

4 carrots

I small red beet

2 celery stalks

I bunch watercress

I bunch spinach

I cucumber

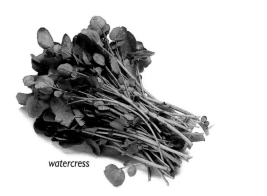

watercress

red beet

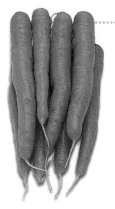

carrot

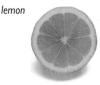

lemon

Sinus Trouble

8 carrots

I tsp fresh horseradish

I lemon, peeled and scraped

(dilute with same amount of water and eat a with spoon over period of two hours)

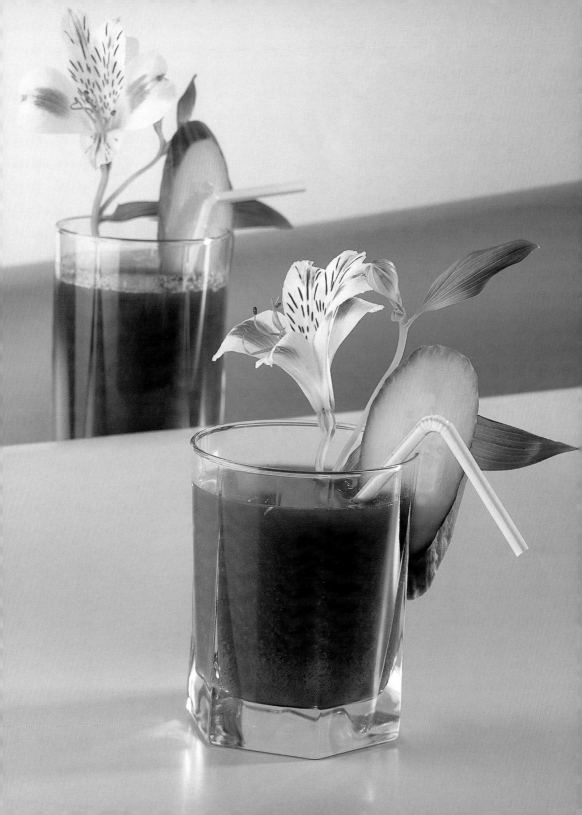

Skin Cleanser

2 raw potatoes

1 green bell pepper

1 cucumber

1 celery stalk or 1 bunch
watercress

watercress

green bell pepper

celery

Water Retention

asparagus

8 asparagus stalks

8 large green and yellow
leaves curly endive

2 celery stalks

1 cucumber

2 carrots

alternatively

¼ watermelon

¼ cantaloupe with seeds

1 lemon, skin scraped

watermelon

endive

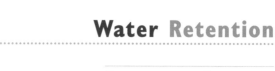

carrot

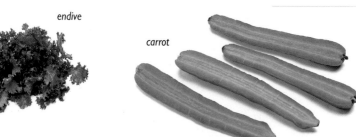

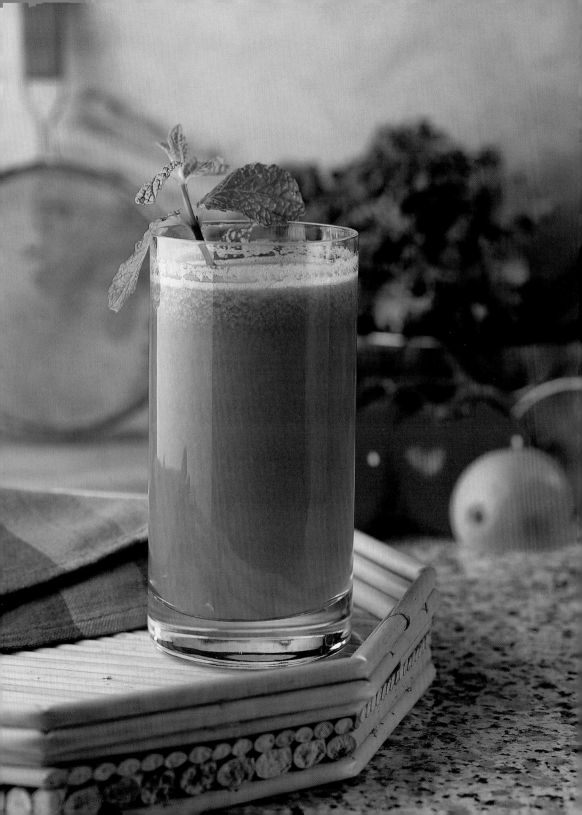

Pomegranate Juice

½ cup pomegranate seeds

½ glass orange juice

Finally, we have a juice that is excellent for a number of conditions including intestinal irritations, high blood pressure and arteriosclerosis.

Remove the pomegranate seeds from the fruit shell and white skin in between.

Balancing Pomegranate Cocktail

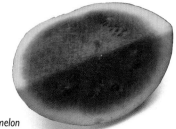

watermelon

seeds from 2 large pomegranates

¼ seedless watermelon

½ cup of lemon or lime juice

2 tbsp honey

2 tbsp chopped fresh mint

Immune-boosting Pomegranate Cocktail

seeds from 2 large pomegranates

4 large carrots

juice from ½ lime

1 tbsp maple syrup

lemon

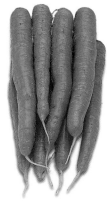

carrot

60

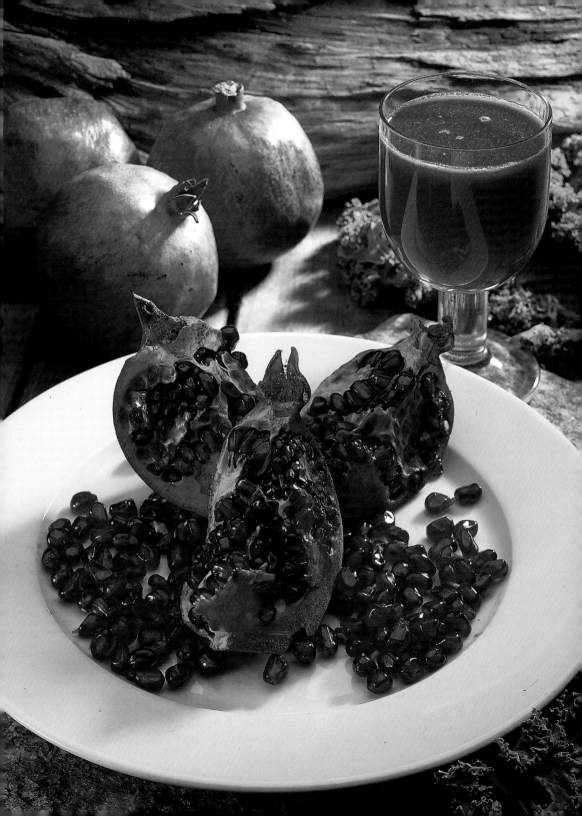

Recipes for Fun and Fitness

The wake-me-upper breakfast

1 grapefruit, outer skin scraped off

1 lemon, outer skin scraped off

2 slices pineapple

¼ honeydew melon

The Tropical Party Punch

If you have guests coming, surprise them with a heavenly punch. I swear it will bring you compliments galore.

6 grapefruits, peel scraped

6 oranges, peel scraped

1 large lime or lemon, peel scraped

1 pineapple, remove skin

1 large papaya

4 passion fruits

The weight-watch-fitness program

Curb your daily food intake to a maximum of 1,150 calories. Replace all refined vegetable oils (supermarket oils), hydrogenated fatty acids (found in vegetable shortening, margarine and hidden in all baked goods and processed packaged foods) with two tablespoons each of the following: unrefined flax oil, pumpkin seed oil, virgin olive oil and butter (no other animal fat). Use the oils in salad dressings or on vegetables. Use olive oil for cooking or sautéing, and butter and cheese on your sandwiches.

Before your meals, drink the following daily cocktail made with:

6 tomatoes

1 red beet with tops

8 carrots

½ head of curly endive or 5 Belgium endive (chicory)

3 celery stalks

1 bunch spinach

1 bunch of watercress or 6 red radishes or 1 black radish

tomato

spinach

orange

Because of the high alkalinity of the weight-watch-fitness program cocktail it will detoxify your system, clearing away a lot of metabolic waste and, as a diuretic, it will help the kidneys expel water. Drink plenty of water or herbal tea during this course, at least 1.5 liters, in addition to the juices. And don't forget to exercise, as trained muscles burn more energy, even while resting.

s o u r c e s

Sources

Flora
7400 Fraser Park drive
Burnaby, BC
V5J 5B9
Tel: (604) 436-6000
1-800-663-0617 (Western Canada)
1-800-387-7541 (Eastern Canada)

Hallelujah Acres
RR #2 Shallow Lake, ON
N0N 2K0
Tel: (519) 935-9999
Fax: (519) 935-3044
PO Box 2038
900 South Post Rd
Shelby, NC 28151

Health Line Naturals
7440 Fraser Park Drive
Burnaby, BC
V5J 5B9

Miracle Exclusive Inc.
64 Seaview Blvd.
Port Washington, NY
11050
Tel: (516) 621-3333
Fax: (516) 621-1997

Nature Clean
Fruit & Veggie Wash
Frank T. Ross & Sons Ltd.
6550 Lawrence Ave. E
Toronto, ON
M1C 4A7

Organika
Para-wash
Organika Health Products Inc.
Richmond, BC
V6V 2H9

Teldon of Canada Ltd.
7432 Fraser Park Drive
Burnaby, BC
V5J 5B9
Order Line: 1-800-663-2212
E-mail: teldon@ultranet.ca

Tribest Corporation
12020 Woodruff Avenue Suite C
Downey, CA
90241
Tel: (562) 935-9999

First published in 2000 by
alive books
7436 Fraser Park Drive
Burnaby BC V5J 5B9
(604) 435–1919
1-800–661–0303

© 2000 by Siegfried Gursche

Book Design:
    Paul Chau
Artwork:
    Terence Yeung
    Raymond Cheung
Food styling:
    Fred Edrissi
Photographs:
    Edmond Fong
Photo Editing:
    Sabine Edrissi-Bredenbrock
Editing:
    Sandra Tonn
    Marian MacLean

Canadian Cataloguing in
Publication Data

Gursche, Siegfried, 1933 -
    Juicing—for the Health of it !

(alive natural health guides, 3
ISSN 1490-6503)
ISBN 1-55312-003-5
Second printing, 2000

Printed in Canada

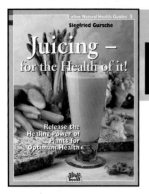

alive Natural Health Guides 3

Siegfried Gursche

Juicing –
for the Health of it!

Release the
Healing Power of
Plants for
Optimum Health

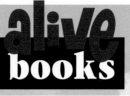

alive books

Natural
Your best source of

We hope you enjoyed **Juicing**.
There are 32 other titles to choose from in *alive*'s library of Natural Health Guides, and more coming soon. The first series of its kind in North America - now sold on 5 continents!

Self-Help Information

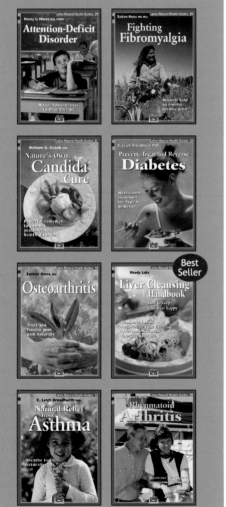

Attention-Deficit Disorder — Nancy L. Morse

Fighting Fibromyalgia — Zoltan Rona MD MSc

Nature's Own Candida Cure — William G. Crook MD

Prevent, Treat and Reverse Diabetes — C. Leigh Broadhurst PhD

Osteoarthritis — Zoltan Rona MD

Liver Cleansing Handbook — Rhody Lake — Best Seller

Natural Relief from Asthma — C. Leigh Broadhurst MD

Rheumatoid Arthritis — Zoltan Rona MD

Healing Foods & Herbs

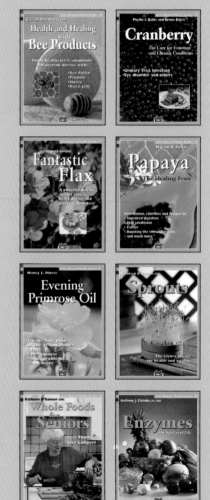

Health and Healing with Bee Products — C. Leigh Broadhurst PhD

Cranberry — Phyllis L. Dales and Bruce Dales

Fantastic Flax — Siegfried Gursche

Papaya — Harald W. Tietze

Evening Primrose Oil — Nancy L. Morse

Sprouts — Kathleen O'Bannon CNC

Whole Foods for Seniors — Kathleen O'Bannon CNC

Enzymes — Anthony J. Cichoke DC MD

expert authors · easy-to-read information · tasty recipes